MW01168502

Low Residue Diet Guide for Beginners

Ensuring Adequate Nutrition on a Low Residue Diet

By

Burke Calum

Table of Contents

CHAPTER 1

Introduction to Low Residue Diet

1.1 Understanding Residue in Foods

The concept of "residue in foods" forms the crux of understanding a low residue diet. Residue refers to undigested or partially digested food material that moves through the digestive tract and ultimately contributes to stool bulk. This undigested matter includes fiber, particularly insoluble fiber, as well as some other components like certain complex carbohydrates and plant matter.

In essence, a low residue diet is specifically designed to minimize the amount and bulk of this undigested material passing through the gastrointestinal system. This reduction in residue helps to decrease the frequency and volume of bowel movements, which can be beneficial for individuals with certain digestive conditions or those recovering from certain medical procedures, such as surgeries involving the gastrointestinal tract.

Foods high in residue typically include whole grains, seeds, nuts, raw fruits, and vegetables. These foods contain significant amounts of fiber, which adds bulk to stool and promotes regular bowel movements. While fiber is generally beneficial for digestive health, in certain situations, reducing its intake becomes necessary to manage symptoms such as diarrhea, abdominal pain, inflammation, or to facilitate healing after surgery.

Understanding the impact of residue in foods involves recognizing that not all fibers are created equal. There are two main types of dietary fiber: soluble and insoluble. Soluble fiber dissolves in water and forms a gel-like substance, slowing down digestion and absorption of nutrients. Insoluble fiber, on the other hand, does not dissolve in water and adds bulk to stool.

A low residue diet typically limits both types of fiber, aiming to reduce the overall fiber content in the diet. It also often restricts other components known to increase stool bulk, such as certain tough skins or membranes in fruits and vegetables. This reduction helps in minimizing bowel movements, alleviating discomfort, and providing the digestive system with a chance to heal, especially in cases of inflammatory bowel disease (IBD), diverticulitis, Crohn's disease, or after surgeries like bowel resections.

It's important to note that adopting a low residue diet should generally be a temporary measure and isn't suitable for everyone. Some individuals, such as those requiring high fiber diets for regular bowel function or certain health conditions like constipation, might not benefit from this dietary approach.

comprehending the role of residue in foods is pivotal when considering a low residue diet. This understanding guides individuals in making informed dietary choices to manage specific digestive issues while ensuring adequate nutrition and promoting gastrointestinal comfort and healing. Consulting with a healthcare professional or a registered dietitian is crucial before starting any significant dietary changes, including adopting a low residue diet, to ensure it aligns with individual health needs and goals.

1.2 Purpose and Benefits of a Low Residue Diet

A low residue diet serves a specific purpose and offers several potential benefits for individuals facing certain digestive challenges or recovering from gastrointestinal procedures. Here are the purposes and benefits elucidating why this dietary approach can be advantageous:

1. Managing Gastrointestinal Symptoms: The primary purpose of a low residue diet is to alleviate symptoms associated with certain gastrointestinal conditions such as inflammatory bowel disease (IBD), Crohn's disease, diverticulitis, ulcerative colitis, or after surgeries involving the digestive tract. By reducing the bulk and frequency of bowel movements, it can help in controlling diarrhea, abdominal cramping, and discomfort, providing relief for individuals experiencing these symptoms.

2. Promoting Bowel Rest: For those recovering from surgery involving the digestive system or experiencing an active flare-up of certain gastrointestinal disorders, a low residue diet offers the digestive tract a period of rest. Minimizing fiber and residue in foods reduces the workload on the intestines, allowing them to heal and recover more effectively.

3. Supporting Healing: By decreasing the volume and frequency of stool, a low residue diet aids in minimizing irritation and inflammation in the intestines. This can be particularly beneficial for individuals with conditions characterized by intestinal inflammation, as it may help in reducing irritation and promoting healing.

4. Providing Symptom Relief: Some individuals with chronic gastrointestinal conditions experience symptoms such as bloating, gas, and abdominal pain due to high-fiber or high-residue foods. Adopting a low residue diet can alleviate these symptoms by reducing the fermentation of fiber in the gut, subsequently decreasing gas production and bloating.

5. Temporary Dietary Management: It serves as a temporary dietary intervention rather than a long-term lifestyle change. Once symptoms are managed or the digestive system has healed, individuals can gradually reintroduce higher fiber foods back into their diet for better overall digestive health.

6. Customization and Adaptability:

Another advantage of a low residue diet is its adaptability and customization. It can be tailored to suit individual needs and tolerances, allowing flexibility in food choices within the limitations of reducing dietary residue.

However, while a low residue diet offers these benefits, it's essential to consider potential drawbacks. Limiting fiber intake for an extended period may lead to deficiencies in certain nutrients found abundantly in high-fiber foods, such as vitamins, minerals, and antioxidants. Therefore, it's crucial to seek guidance from a healthcare professional or a registered dietitian to ensure that the diet remains nutritionally adequate while meeting specific digestive needs.

1.3 Who Might Benefit from a Low Residue Diet

A low residue diet can be beneficial for several groups of individuals who experience specific gastrointestinal challenges or require temporary dietary modifications. Here's a breakdown of who might benefit from adopting a low residue diet:

1. Individuals with Inflammatory Bowel Disease (IBD): Those with Crohn's disease or ulcerative colitis often experience flare-ups characterized by abdominal pain, diarrhea, and inflammation in the intestines. A low residue diet can help manage symptoms during these periods by reducing bowel movements and minimizing irritation in the gut.

2. Post-Surgery Patients: After gastrointestinal surgeries like bowel resections or surgeries involving the colon, adopting a low residue diet can aid in the healing process. It allows the digestive tract time to recover by reducing the workload and minimizing stool volume, promoting faster recovery and reducing potential complications.

3. Diverticulitis Patients: During acute episodes of diverticulitis, where pouches in the colon become inflamed or infected, a low residue diet can alleviate symptoms by easing the passage of stool through the affected area, reducing strain on the colon walls, and allowing inflammation to subside.

4. Individuals with Digestive Disorders: Some individuals with specific digestive disorders or sensitivities, such as irritable bowel syndrome (IBS) or bowel strictures, might find relief from symptoms like abdominal cramping, bloating, and diarrhea by adopting a low residue diet.

5. Patients Undergoing Radiation Therapy: For individuals undergoing radiation therapy targeting the abdomen or pelvic area, a low residue diet might be recommended to minimize bowel movements and reduce irritation in the intestines, easing discomfort during treatment.

6. Short-Term Symptom Management:
In certain situations where individuals experience temporary gastrointestinal distress, such as acute diarrhea, abdominal pain, or excessive gas, a short-term adoption of a low residue diet can provide relief until symptoms subside.

7. Preparation for Medical Procedures:
Prior to certain medical procedures like colonoscopies or imaging tests involving the gastrointestinal tract, a temporary shift to a low residue diet may be advised to clear the digestive system and improve visualization during the procedure.

However, it's crucial to emphasize that a low residue diet isn't a one-size-fits-all solution. Not everyone with a gastrointestinal issue benefit from or requires this dietary approach. Some individuals, like those needing high fiber for regular bowel function or specific health conditions like constipation, might not find this diet suitable.

Ultimately, the decision to adopt a low residue diet should be made in consultation with a healthcare professional or a registered dietitian who can evaluate an individual's specific health needs, consider the potential benefits and drawbacks, and tailor dietary recommendations accordingly.

CHAPTER 2

Fundamentals of a Low Residue Diet

2.1 What is a Low Residue Diet?

A low residue diet is a specific eating plan designed to reduce the amount of undigested or partially digested food material (residue) passing through the gastrointestinal tract. This dietary approach restricts foods that are high in fiber and other components known to contribute to stool bulk, aiming to minimize the volume and frequency of bowel movements.

The key characteristics of a low residue diet include:

1. Limited Fiber Content: It significantly reduces the intake of dietary fiber, both soluble and insoluble. Fiber-rich foods such as whole grains, seeds, nuts, raw fruits, and vegetables are restricted or consumed in limited quantities.

2. Emphasis on Low-Residue Foods: The diet focuses on consuming easily digestible and low-residue foods that are less likely to contribute to stool bulk. This includes refined grains, cooked and peeled fruits and vegetables, well-cooked lean proteins, and certain processed foods.

3. Avoidance of Certain Foods: High-fiber foods, roughage, seeds, skins, and tough membranes present in certain fruits and vegetables are generally avoided. Additionally, foods that tend to increase gas production or fermentation in the gut, such as beans and certain dairy products, might also be limited.

4. Processed and Refined Foods: The diet may include more processed or refined food options, such as white bread, refined pasta, and strained fruit juices, as these tend to have lower fiber content and are easier to digest.

5. Modification of Food Preparation: Cooking methods like peeling, deseeding, and thorough cooking of fruits and vegetables are often recommended to reduce their fiber content and make them easier to digest.

6. Adequate Fluid Intake: Maintaining proper hydration is essential, as reducing fiber intake might also decrease the amount of water retained in the stool. Consuming adequate fluids helps prevent constipation and maintains bowel regularity.

7. Individual Customization: A low residue diet can be tailored to meet individual needs, as some people may tolerate certain foods better than others. Customization ensures that the diet remains manageable and nutritionally adequate for the individual's health requirements.

This dietary approach is often recommended for individuals experiencing gastrointestinal symptoms such as diarrhea, abdominal pain, inflammation, or those recovering from surgeries involving the digestive tract. However, it's important to note that a low residue diet is typically considered a short-term intervention rather than a long-term dietary pattern, as prolonged restriction of fiber-rich foods may lead to nutritional deficiencies if not managed properly.

Before starting a low residue diet, consulting with a healthcare professional or a registered dietitian is crucial to ensure that it aligns with an individual's specific health needs and to prevent any potential nutritional imbalances.

2.2 Guidelines and Principles

Here are the fundamental guidelines and principles for following a low residue diet:

1. Limit High-Fiber Foods: Avoid or limit foods high in fiber, such as whole grains, bran, seeds, nuts, raw fruits, and vegetables. opt for refined or processed alternatives with lower fiber content.

2. Choose Refined Grains: Select refined grains and products made from refined flours, such as white bread, white rice, and refined pasta, over their whole grain counterparts to reduce fiber intake.

3. Cook and Peel Fruits and Vegetables: Prioritize cooked, peeled, or canned fruits and vegetables, as they tend to have lower fiber content compared to raw ones. Removing skins, seeds, and tough parts further reduces residue.

4. Avoid Certain Fruits and Vegetables: Steer clear of high-residue fruits and vegetables, including berries, citrus fruits with membranes, raw leafy greens, broccoli, cauliflower, and beans.

5. Opt for Well-Cooked Proteins: Choose lean, well-cooked meats, poultry, fish, eggs, and tofu as protein sources, avoiding tough or fibrous cuts of meat that may be harder to digest.

6. Use Low-Fiber Dairy: Consume low-lactose or lactose-free dairy options, like lactose-free milk, yogurt without seeds or fruit chunks, and mild cheeses.

7. Be Mindful of Added Fiber: Check food labels and avoid products fortified with extra fiber or whole grains.

8. Control Portion Sizes: Even with low residue foods, moderation is key. Eating smaller, frequent meals throughout the day can help manage symptoms.

9. Stay Hydrated: Drink plenty of fluids, especially water, to prevent constipation and maintain proper hydration, as reducing fiber intake can impact stool consistency.

10. Individualize the Diet: Modify the diet based on personal tolerance and preferences. Some foods may affect individuals differently, so customizing the diet helps manage symptoms effectively.

11. Gradual Transition: When transitioning to or from a low residue diet, do it gradually to allow the digestive system time to adapt and minimize any discomfort.

12. Consult a Healthcare Professional: Before starting or making significant changes to a low residue diet, seek guidance from a healthcare professional or a registered dietitian. They can provide tailored advice and ensure that the diet meets individual nutritional needs while managing specific health concerns.

Adhering to these guidelines helps reduce the volume and frequency of bowel movements, alleviating gastrointestinal symptoms and providing the digestive system with a chance to heal. However, it's important to remember that a low residue diet is typically a short-term intervention and should be used under the guidance of a healthcare professional to prevent potential nutritional deficiencies and ensure overall health.

2.3 Differences from Other Diets (Low Fiber, Low FODMAP, etc.)

While certain dietary approaches might seem similar, there are distinct differences between a low residue diet and other diets like low fiber diets, low FODMAP diets, and others targeting gastrointestinal health. Here's an overview of how they differ:

1. Low Residue Diet vs. Low Fiber Diet:

- **Low Residue Diet:** Primarily focuses on minimizing the overall amount of undigested or partially digested food material (residue) passing through the gastrointestinal tract. It restricts high-fiber foods, both soluble and insoluble, to reduce stool bulk and frequency.

- **Low Fiber Diet:** Generally reduces the intake of dietary fiber but doesn't necessarily restrict residue. It's often used to manage symptoms of gastrointestinal conditions or after certain surgeries, but the emphasis isn't solely on minimizing residue. Some high-residue foods might be allowed in limited quantities.

2. Low Residue Diet vs. Low FODMAP Diet:

- **Low Residue Diet:** Aims to decrease the bulk and frequency of bowel movements by limiting high-fiber foods. It's mainly focused on reducing residue to manage symptoms like diarrhea, abdominal pain, and inflammation in specific gastrointestinal conditions or during recovery from surgeries.

- **Low FODMAP Diet:** Targets fermentable carbohydrates (FODMAPs) found in certain foods that can trigger digestive symptoms like bloating, gas, and abdominal discomfort. This diet aims to reduce FODMAP intake rather than solely focusing on fiber or residue content. It's often used to manage symptoms of irritable bowel syndrome (IBS) and other functional gastrointestinal disorders.

3. Low Residue Diet vs. Specific Carbohydrate Diet (SCD):

- **Low Residue Diet:** Primarily focused on reducing residue by limiting high-fiber foods to ease the workload on the digestive system and promote healing, particularly after surgeries or during flare-ups of certain gastrointestinal conditions.

- **Specific Carbohydrate Diet:** Restricts specific types of carbohydrates including grains, certain sugars, and complex carbohydrates. It's designed to manage conditions like Crohn's disease, ulcerative colitis, and celiac disease by reducing inflammation and promoting gut healing.

4. Low Residue Diet vs. Elemental Diet:

- **Low Residue Diet:** Involves consuming whole foods, albeit with reduced fiber content. It aims to minimize residue but still allows for a variety of food choices within the limitations of reducing fiber intake.

- **Elemental Diet:** Involves consuming pre-digested nutrients in liquid form. It's often used as a complete meal replacement for individuals with severe digestive disorders or those who require complete bowel rest, providing easily absorbable nutrients without residue.

These dietary approaches have different focuses, mechanisms, and applications in managing various gastrointestinal conditions. Each diet addresses specific aspects of digestion, symptoms, and nutritional intake, tailored to individual needs under the guidance of healthcare professionals or registered dietitians.

CHAPTER 3

Foods to Include in a Low Residue Diet

3.1 Recommended Food Groups and Choices

In a low residue diet, the focus is on consuming easily digestible foods that are low in fiber and tend to produce minimal waste or residue in the digestive tract. Here are some recommended food groups and choices:

1. Refined Grains and Starches:

- White bread (without seeds or nuts)

- Refined pasta

- White rice

- Plain crackers and refined cereals (avoid those with added seeds or bran)

2. Well-Cooked Vegetables (Peeled and Seedless):

- Peeled and cooked potatoes

- Cooked carrots

- Skinless and seedless squash

- Green beans without strings

- Cooked zucchini or yellow squash

3. Cooked Fruits (Peeled and Seedless):

- Peeled and cooked apples

- Peeled and cooked pears

- Canned fruits in syrup (without skins or seeds)

- Applesauce without added skins or seeds

4. Lean Proteins:

- Well-cooked poultry without skin

- Tender cuts of beef or pork without gristle

- Fish without bones

- Eggs prepared without added fat (boiled, poached, or scrambled)

5. Dairy (Low-Lactose Options):

- Lactose-free milk

- Mild cheeses (avoid those with added seeds or nuts)

- Plain yogurt without fruit chunks or seeds

6. Refined Fats and Oils:

- Butter or margarine

- Vegetable oils (such as canola or sunflower oil)

- Mayonnaise without seeds or nuts

7. Beverages:

- Clear juices without pulp (apple juice, strained citrus juices)

- Clear broth or strained soups (avoid those with large amounts of vegetables or grains)

- Water and herbal teas

8. Desserts and Sweets:

- Plain gelatin

- Hard candies and sweets without nuts or seeds

- Marshmallows

These food choices are typically easier to digest and are less likely to contribute to stool bulk or gastrointestinal irritation. Cooking methods like peeling, deseeding, and thorough cooking of fruits and vegetables are essential to reduce their fiber content and make them more suitable for a low residue diet.

However, individual tolerance can vary, so it's important to pay attention to how different foods affect digestive comfort and symptoms. Consulting a healthcare professional or a registered dietitian is recommended to personalize food choices and ensure adequate nutrition while following a low residue diet.

3.2 Meal Planning and Preparation Tips

Here are some meal planning and preparation tips tailored for a low residue diet:

1. Plan Balanced Meals:

- Aim for a balance of protein, carbohydrates, and fats in each meal to ensure adequate nutrition.

- Incorporate low residue foods from different food groups to diversify your diet.

2. Portion Control:

- Opt for smaller, more frequent meals throughout the day to avoid overwhelming the digestive system.

- Avoid large meals, which might trigger discomfort or excessive bowel movements.

3. Food Preparation Techniques:

- Peel and deseed fruits and vegetables before cooking or consuming to reduce their fiber content.

- Cook foods thoroughly and opt for softer textures to make them easier to digest.

4. Experiment with Cooking Methods:

- Choose cooking methods like boiling, steaming, or stewing to soften foods and break down fiber.

- Consider pureeing or blending foods to create smoother textures, especially for fruits and vegetables.

5. Incorporate Low Residue Proteins:

- Focus on lean and well-cooked proteins like poultry, fish, eggs, and tender cuts of meat without tough connective tissue.

6. Use Refined Grains:

- Substitute refined grains such as white bread, pasta, and rice for their whole grain counterparts to lower fiber intake.

7. Meal Ideas:

- Breakfast: Plain oatmeal made with refined oats, scrambled eggs, white toast, and peeled, cooked apples.

- Lunch: Chicken or turkey sandwich on white bread, with peeled cucumber slices and a low-fiber fruit like peeled grapes.

- Dinner: Baked fish or chicken breast, well-cooked carrots and squash, and white rice.

8. Be Mindful of Seasonings and Sauces:

- Avoid spicy or heavily seasoned foods that might irritate the digestive system.

- Use mild seasonings and limit the use of high-fiber herbs and spices.

9. Hydration is Key:

- Drink plenty of fluids, especially water, to prevent dehydration and aid digestion.

10. Keep a Food Journal:

- Track the foods you eat and how they affect your symptoms to identify triggers or intolerances.

11. Gradual Transition:

- When transitioning onto or off of a low residue diet, do it gradually to allow your digestive system time to adjust.

12. Seek Professional Guidance:

- Consult with a healthcare professional or a registered dietitian to create a personalized meal plan that meets your nutritional needs while managing symptoms.

Adapting these meal planning and preparation strategies can help in maintaining a varied and nutritious diet while effectively managing symptoms associated with a low residue diet. Customizing meal plans according to individual preferences and tolerances is key to finding the right balance between comfort and nutritional adequacy.

3.3 Recipe Ideas and Sample Menus

here are some recipe ideas and sample menus suitable for a low residue diet:

Sample Menu Ideas:

Breakfast:

- Scrambled eggs with low-fat cheese

- White toast or a refined bagel

- Peeled and cooked apples or applesauce

- Lactose-free yogurt

Lunch:

- Turkey or chicken sandwich on white bread with lettuce (well-washed and dried) and peeled cucumber slices

- Clear broth-based soup with well-cooked vegetables (strained)

- Low-fiber fruit like peeled and sliced melon

Dinner:

- Baked or grilled fish (without skin) with lemon

- Mashed potatoes (without skins) or well-cooked white rice

- Cooked carrots and green beans

- Gelatin dessert or peeled, cooked pears

Recipe Ideas:

1. Lemon Herb Baked Chicken:

- Ingredients:

    - Boneless, skinless chicken breasts

    - Lemon juice

    - Herbs like parsley, thyme, and rosemary

    - Salt and pepper

- Instructions:

    - Marinate chicken breasts in lemon juice and herbs.

    - Bake until fully cooked and tender.

2. Easy Vegetable Soup:

- Ingredients:

    - Low-residue vegetables like carrots, green beans, and peeled potatoes

    - Low-sodium chicken or vegetable broth

    - Salt and pepper for seasoning

- Instructions:

    - Chop vegetables into small pieces.

    - Simmer in broth until vegetables are soft.

    - Season to taste with salt and pepper.

3. Baked White Fish with Herbs:

- Ingredients:

    - White fish fillets (such as cod or tilapia)

- Fresh herbs like parsley and dill

- Lemon slices

- Olive oil

- Instructions:

    - Place fish fillets on a baking sheet.

    - Drizzle with olive oil, top with herbs and lemon slices.

    - Bake until the fish is cooked through and flakes easily.

4. Creamy Mashed Potatoes:

- Ingredients:

    - Peeled and boiled potatoes

    - Butter or lactose-free margarine

    - Milk or lactose-free milk

    - Salt and pepper

- Instructions:

    - Mash boiled potatoes with butter and milk until creamy.

    - Season with salt and pepper to taste.

5. Fruit Compote:

- Ingredients:

    - Peeled and diced apples or pears

    - Cinnamon

    - Water or apple juice

    - Optional: a touch of honey

- Instructions:

    - Simmer diced fruits with water or apple juice until soft.

- Add cinnamon and honey if desired, then cool before serving.

These recipes and menu ideas focus on using low-residue, easily digestible ingredients while ensuring meals remain flavorful and satisfying. Adjust seasonings and ingredients to suit individual taste preferences and dietary requirements. Always consult with a healthcare professional or a registered dietitian for personalized advice on adapting recipes to meet specific nutritional needs.

CHAPTER 4

Foods to Avoid on a Low Residue Diet

4.1 High Residue Foods to Steer Clear Off

Here's a list of high-residue foods that are typically avoided or limited on a low residue diet:

1. Whole Grains:

- Whole grain bread and rolls

- Whole wheat pasta

- Brown rice

- Whole grain cereals with added bran or seeds

2. Seeds and Nuts:

- Chia seeds

- Flaxseeds

- Sunflower seeds

- Almonds, walnuts, pecans, and other nuts

3. Raw Fruits and Vegetables:

- Raw apples and pears (with skins)

- Berries (strawberries, raspberries, etc.)

- Raw carrots

- Broccoli and cauliflower

- Raw leafy greens (spinach, kale, lettuce)

4. High-Fiber Legumes:

- Beans (kidney beans, black beans, lentils)

- Peas

- Chickpeas

5. Tough Skins and Membranes:

- Citrus fruits with membranes (orange, grapefruit)

- Fruits and vegetables with tough skins (kiwi, grapes)

- Tough vegetable skins (potato skins)

6. High-Fiber Dairy:

- Dairy products with added seeds or nuts (some specialty cheeses)

- Yogurts with fruit chunks or seeds

- Full-fat milk

7. High-Fiber Snacks and Condiments:

- Granola bars and high-fiber snack bars

- Popcorn

- Salsa with seeds and chunks of vegetables

- High-fiber condiments like mustard with seeds

8. Spices and High-Fiber Herbs:

- Spicy seasonings that might irritate the digestive tract

- High-fiber herbs and spices (like cumin seeds)

9. Other High-Residue Foods:

- Bran-based cereals and muffins

- Coconut

- Dried fruits with skins (raisins, apricots)

Avoiding these high-residue foods helps reduce the fiber content and decreases the volume and frequency of bowel movements. It aims to alleviate symptoms associated with specific gastrointestinal conditions or during recovery from surgeries. However, individual tolerances may vary, so it's essential to monitor how different foods affect digestive comfort and symptoms. Consulting a healthcare professional or a registered dietitian for personalized guidance is recommended when following a low residue diet.

4.2 Common Mistakes to Avoid

When following a low residue diet, certain common mistakes can hinder its effectiveness or lead to unintended consequences. Here are some key mistakes to avoid:

1. Not Gradually Transitioning:
Abruptly changing to a low residue diet can shock the digestive system. Gradually transition by slowly reducing high-residue foods to allow your body to adjust.

2. Overlooking Nutritional Balance:
Focusing solely on reducing residue might lead to nutritional deficiencies. Ensure your diet includes a variety of nutrient-rich foods to meet your body's needs.

3. Ignoring Fluid Intake: Forgetting to maintain adequate hydration can exacerbate constipation. Drink plenty of fluids to prevent dehydration and help maintain regularity.

4. Relying Heavily on Processed Foods: Depending too much on processed or refined foods can compromise overall nutritional quality. Aim for a balance between processed options and whole, low-residue foods.

5. Not Paying Attention to Portion Sizes: Even low-residue foods can cause discomfort if consumed in large quantities. Control portion sizes to avoid overwhelming the digestive system.

6. Cutting Out Fiber Completely: While the goal is to reduce fiber intake, eliminating it entirely can lead to other digestive issues. Work with a healthcare professional to find a suitable balance for your specific needs.

7. Not Monitoring Symptoms and Adjusting: Failing to track how different foods affect your symptoms can hinder

your ability to manage your diet
effectively. Keep a food journal and note
any reactions to foods.

8. Neglecting Professional Guidance:
Avoiding consultations with healthcare
professionals or registered dietitians can
result in improper dietary adjustments or
inadequate nutrition. Seek professional
guidance for personalized advice.

9. Overlooking Food Preparation
Techniques: Incorrectly preparing low-
residue foods by not peeling, deseeding, or
cooking them thoroughly can inadvertently
increase their fiber content.

10. Sticking to the Diet Longer Than
Necessary: Prolonging a low residue diet
beyond its intended period can lead to
nutritional deficiencies. Gradually
reintroduce higher fiber foods when
symptoms improve or as advised by your
healthcare provider.

Being mindful of these mistakes and
taking steps to avoid them can contribute

to a more effective and balanced approach to managing symptoms while following a low residue diet. Remember, individual tolerances and needs can vary, so seeking professional guidance ensures the diet aligns with your health requirements.

4.3 Hidden Sources of Residue

Even when following a low residue diet, some foods or ingredients may contain hidden sources of residue. Here are some common hidden sources to be cautious of:

1. Processed Foods:

- Some processed foods may contain hidden high-fiber ingredients like whole grains, bran, or seeds. Check labels for added fibers or whole grains.

2. Condiments and Sauces:

- Certain condiments or sauces may contain seeds or high-fiber ingredients. Mustard, relish, and some salad dressings might have seeds or vegetable chunks.

3. Canned or Prepackaged Meals:

- Ready-made canned or prepackaged meals may contain ingredients that contribute to residue. Always check labels for fiber content.

4. Medications and Supplements:

- Some medications or supplements might contain fillers or binding agents that could be high in fiber. Discuss alternatives with your healthcare provider if needed.

5. Low-Fiber Foods in Excessive Amounts:

- Consuming large quantities of even low-fiber foods can inadvertently increase residue. Control portion sizes to avoid overconsumption.

6. Unpeeled or Unprocessed "Low Residue" Foods:

- Certain low-residue foods may still contain fiber if they're unpeeled or not properly processed. Ensure fruits, vegetables, and grains are appropriately prepared.

7. Dairy Products with Hidden Fiber Additions:

- Some flavored or processed dairy products may contain added fiber sources. opt for plain versions or carefully read labels for added ingredients.

8. Restaurant or Takeout Meals:

- Foods from restaurants or takeout might have hidden high-residue ingredients. Request simple, customized options when dining out.

9. Snacks and Baked Goods:

- Snack bars, baked goods, or cookies may contain added fibers, seeds, or whole grains. Choose carefully and check labels.

10. Unstrained or Unfiltered Beverages:

- Certain beverages, especially those with pulp or seeds, might contain residue. Opt for clear juices without pulp or herbal teas.

Being mindful of these hidden sources of residue can help maintain the effectiveness of a low residue diet. Reading food labels, preparing meals at home using low-residue ingredients, and being cautious when dining out or consuming packaged foods can assist in reducing unintended intake of high-residue substances. Consulting with a healthcare professional or a registered dietitian for guidance on navigating hidden sources of residue can be beneficial.

CHAPTER 5

Managing Nutritional Balance

5.1 Ensuring Adequate Nutrition on a Low Residue Diet

Maintaining adequate nutrition on a low residue diet is crucial, despite the restrictions on certain foods. Here are ways to ensure nutritional balance:

1. Include Low-Residue Nutrient-Dense Foods:

- Choose nutrient-rich, low-residue options such as peeled and cooked fruits, well-cooked vegetables, lean proteins, and refined grains to ensure adequate intake of essential nutrients.

2. Focus on Protein Sources:

- Prioritize lean proteins like poultry, fish, eggs, and tofu to meet protein requirements for tissue repair and overall health.

3. Incorporate Good Fats:

- Include healthy fats from sources like olive oil, avocados, and nuts in moderate amounts to support nutrient absorption and overall health.

4. Fortify Foods with Nutrient Additions:

- Consider fortified foods or supplements recommended by healthcare professionals to compensate for potential nutrient deficiencies due to dietary restrictions.

5. Use Nutrient-Rich Cooking Methods:

- Opt for cooking methods that retain nutrients, like steaming or lightly boiling vegetables, to minimize nutrient loss during food preparation.

6. Consume Small, Frequent Meals:

- Eating smaller, frequent meals can aid in better nutrient absorption and digestion, allowing the body to utilize nutrients effectively.

7. Monitor and Supplement if Necessary:

- Monitor nutrient levels through regular check-ups and blood tests. If deficiencies arise, consider targeted supplementation under healthcare provider guidance.

8. Emphasize Hydration:

- Ensure adequate hydration to support digestion and overall health. Consume water, clear juices, and herbal teas throughout the day.

9. Gradual Reintroduction of Foods:

- Once symptoms subside or as advised by healthcare professionals, gradually reintroduce higher-fiber foods to ensure a more balanced diet.

10. Consult a Registered Dietitian:

- Seek guidance from a registered dietitian to create a customized meal plan that meets individual nutritional needs while managing symptoms effectively.

Balancing nutritional needs while following a low residue diet requires careful planning and consideration of nutrient-rich, easily digestible options. Monitoring symptoms, regularly assessing nutritional status, and seeking professional guidance play key roles in ensuring adequate nutrition during dietary restrictions.

5.2 Potential Nutrient Deficiencies and How to Address Them

A Low Residue Diet, while beneficial for certain medical conditions, may pose challenges in terms of obtaining a well-rounded spectrum of nutrients. By limiting high-fiber foods, individuals following this diet may be at risk of deficiencies in essential vitamins and minerals. Here are some potential nutrient deficiencies and strategies to address them:

1. **Fiber Deficiency:**

- *Risk:* Since a Low Residue Diet restricts fiber intake, there's a risk of insufficient dietary fiber, which is crucial for digestive health.

- *Addressing the Deficiency:*

    - Incorporate soluble fiber sources such as oats, psyllium husk, and fruits like bananas.

- Consider fiber supplements under the guidance of a healthcare professional.

2. **Vitamin D Deficiency:**

- *Risk:* Limited exposure to sunlight and a reduced intake of vitamin D-rich foods can lead to deficiencies.

- *Addressing the Deficiency:*

    - Include vitamin D-fortified foods like fortified dairy or plant-based milk.

    - Discuss supplementation with a healthcare provider to ensure adequate levels.

3. **Calcium Deficiency:**

- *Risk:* Dairy products, a common source of calcium, may be restricted. Calcium is vital for bone health.

- *Addressing the Deficiency:*

- Explore non-dairy sources like fortified plant milk, leafy greens, and canned fish with bones.

- Consider calcium supplements, especially if dietary intake is insufficient.

4. **Iron Deficiency:**

- *Risk:* Reducing high-residue foods may impact iron absorption. Iron is essential for preventing anemia.

- *Addressing the Deficiency:*

    - Consume lean meats, poultry, fish, and iron-fortified cereals.

    - Pair iron-rich foods with vitamin C sources to enhance absorption.

5. **B Vitamins (B6, B12, Folate) Deficiency:**

- *Risk:* Limited intake of certain grains and fortified cereals may contribute to B vitamin deficiencies.

- *Addressing the Deficiency:*

    - Include B vitamin-rich foods like lean meats, eggs, and fortified grains.

    - Consider B complex supplements, especially if there are absorption concerns.

6. **Potassium Deficiency:**

- *Risk:* Restricting high-potassium foods like bananas and potatoes may lead to deficiencies.

- *Addressing the Deficiency:*

    - Include low-residue sources of potassium like melons and canned fruits.

- Consult with a healthcare professional for guidance on potassium supplements.

7. **Magnesium Deficiency:**

- *Risk:* Limited intake of whole grains and legumes may impact magnesium levels.

- *Addressing the Deficiency:*

  - Consume magnesium-rich foods such as nuts, seeds, and green leafy vegetables.

  - Discuss magnesium supplements with a healthcare provider if needed.

8. **Protein Deficiency:**

- *Risk:* A reduced intake of high-fiber plant sources may affect protein intake.

- *Addressing the Deficiency:*

- Include lean meats, poultry, fish, eggs, and dairy products.

- Consider protein supplements if dietary protein is insufficient.

It's crucial for individuals on a Low Residue Diet to work closely with healthcare professionals, including dietitians, to monitor nutrient levels and make necessary adjustments to ensure a balanced and nutritious diet. Regular check-ups and tailored dietary plans can help mitigate the risk of nutrient deficiencies and promote overall well-being.

5.3 Supplements and Their Role

Supplements play a crucial role in supporting individuals on a Low Residue Diet by addressing potential nutrient gaps and ensuring optimal health. While it's essential to obtain nutrients from whole foods whenever possible, certain circumstances may necessitate supplementation. Here's an exploration of common supplements and their roles in the context of a Low Residue Diet:

1. **Multivitamins:**

- *Role:* Multivitamins can provide a broad spectrum of essential vitamins and minerals, acting as a nutritional safety net.

- *Considerations:* Choose a multivitamin tailored to individual needs, and consult with a healthcare professional to avoid excessive intake of specific nutrients.

2. **Fiber Supplements:**

- *Role:* In cases where fiber intake is restricted, soluble fiber supplements like psyllium husk can help support digestive health.

- *Considerations:* Introduce fiber supplements gradually to prevent digestive discomfort, and stay adequately hydrated to support their effectiveness.

3. **Calcium Supplements:**

- *Role:* Essential for bone health, calcium supplements can be considered if dietary intake is insufficient due to limitations on dairy products.

- *Considerations:* Opt for calcium citrate, which is more easily absorbed, and discuss dosage with a healthcare provider to prevent excess intake.

4. **Vitamin D Supplements:**

- *Role:* Particularly important for individuals with limited sun exposure, vitamin D supplements contribute to bone health.

- *Considerations:* Regular monitoring of vitamin D levels is recommended, and supplementation should be done under healthcare guidance.

5. Iron Supplements:

- *Role:* Addressing the risk of iron deficiency, supplements can be beneficial, especially for individuals with limited intake of iron-rich foods.

- *Considerations:* Consult with a healthcare provider to determine the appropriate type and dosage of iron supplements to avoid side effects.

6. B Vitamin Complex:

- *Role:* Essential for energy metabolism, a B vitamin complex can help prevent deficiencies associated with limited intake of certain foods.

- *Considerations:* Tailor supplementation based on individual needs, and discuss with healthcare professionals to ensure an appropriate balance of B vitamins.

7. **Potassium and Magnesium Supplements:**

- *Role:* In cases where dietary potassium and magnesium are restricted, supplements can help maintain electrolyte balance.

- *Considerations:* Regular monitoring of blood levels is essential, and supplementation should be guided by healthcare professionals to prevent excess intake.

8. **Protein Supplements:**

- *Role:* Supporting protein intake, especially when high-fiber plant sources are limited, protein supplements can help meet nutritional needs.

- *Considerations:* Choose high-quality protein supplements, and use them as a complement to, not a replacement for, dietary protein sources.

It's paramount for individuals following a Low Residue Diet to coordinate with healthcare providers, including dietitians and physicians, before initiating any supplementation. Regular monitoring, adjustments based on individual needs, and a holistic approach to nutrition are key to ensuring that supplements contribute positively to overall health and well-being. Always seek professional guidance to create a personalized supplement plan tailored to specific dietary restrictions and health goals.

CHAPTER 6

Adapting the Diet to Specific Needs

6.1 Low Residue Diet for Medical Conditions

Adapting a Low Residue Diet to specific medical conditions requires a nuanced approach, considering individual health needs, symptoms, and treatment goals.

1. **Inflammatory Bowel Disease (IBD):**

- *Rationale:* A Low Residue Diet is often recommended during flare-ups of Crohn's disease or ulcerative colitis to reduce gastrointestinal irritation.

- *Adaptations:*

- Gradually reintroduce high-fiber foods during remission.

- Monitor symptoms closely and adjust the diet in consultation with a healthcare provider.

2. **Diverticulitis:**

- *Rationale:* A Low Residue Diet may be prescribed during acute episodes to minimize strain on the digestive system.

- *Adaptations:*

  - Transition to a regular diet gradually after symptoms subside.

  - Emphasize fiber-rich foods to prevent future flare-ups during the recovery phase.

3. **Gastrointestinal Surgery:**

- *Rationale:* After certain surgeries, such as bowel resection, a Low Residue Diet is often recommended to allow the digestive tract to heal.

- *Adaptations:*

  - Follow post-surgery dietary guidelines provided by healthcare professionals.

  - Gradually reintroduce foods based on individual tolerance and healing progress.

4. **Radiation or Chemotherapy:**

- *Rationale:* Patients undergoing cancer treatments may experience digestive issues, making a Low Residue Diet beneficial.

- *Adaptations:*

  - Coordinate with oncology and nutrition specialists to ensure adequate nutrition.

- Consider supplementation to address nutrient deficiencies.

5. Short Bowel Syndrome:

- *Rationale:* Individuals with a shortened small intestine may benefit from a Low Residue Diet to reduce the load on the digestive system.

- *Adaptations:*

    - Optimize nutrient absorption through careful food choices.

    - Consider small, frequent meals to support digestion.

6. Chronic Diarrhea or Malabsorption Disorders:

- *Rationale:* Conditions like celiac disease or chronic diarrhea may warrant a Low Residue Diet to manage symptoms.

- *Adaptations:*

    - Emphasize easily digestible and well-tolerated foods.

    - Monitor nutritional status and adjust the diet as needed.

7. **Post-Operative Care:**

- *Rationale:* After abdominal surgeries, a Low Residue Diet may be prescribed to minimize strain on the healing digestive system.

- *Adaptations:*

    - Gradually transition to a regular diet under the guidance of healthcare professionals.

    - Focus on nutrient-dense foods to support recovery.

8. **Individualized Approaches:**

- *Rationale:* Each medical condition and individual response to a Low Residue Diet can vary.

- *Adaptations:*

  - Collaborate with healthcare providers, including dietitians, to create a customized plan.

  - Regularly assess symptoms and make adjustments as needed.

It's crucial for individuals with specific medical conditions to work closely with healthcare professionals to tailor a Low Residue Diet to their unique needs. Regular monitoring, open communication, and adjustments based on health status are key components of a successful dietary management strategy. Always seek personalized guidance to ensure that the adapted diet aligns with both medical requirements and individual preferences.

6.2 Transitioning On and Off the Low Residue Diet

Transitioning onto and off a Low Residue Diet requires careful planning to ensure a smooth adjustment while meeting nutritional needs. Whether it's adapting to a medical recommendation or transitioning back to a regular diet,

1. Transitioning Onto the Low Residue Diet:

- **Gradual Adjustment:**

  - Start by gradually reducing high-fiber foods to minimize sudden changes in bowel habits.

  - Allow the digestive system time to adapt to the lower residue intake.

- **Identify Well-Tolerated Foods:**

  - Introduce easily digestible, low-residue foods such as

white rice, lean proteins, and peeled fruits.

- Monitor individual responses to identify well-tolerated options.

- **Fluid Intake:**

  - Ensure adequate hydration to prevent constipation, especially if fiber intake is reduced.

  - Include clear fluids and broths to maintain hydration levels.

- **Monitor Symptoms:**

  - Regularly assess digestive symptoms and adjust the diet accordingly.

  - Collaborate with healthcare professionals to address any challenges or concerns.

- **Nutrient Optimization:**

- Focus on nutrient-dense foods to meet essential nutritional requirements.

- Consider supplements under the guidance of healthcare providers to address potential deficiencies.

2. **Living on the Low Residue Diet:**

- **Meal Planning:**

    - Plan well-balanced meals with a variety of low-residue options.

    - Explore creative ways to add flavor and variety within the diet restrictions.

- **Regular Monitoring:**

    - Stay vigilant to changes in symptoms and bowel habits.

    - Keep a food diary to track responses to different foods.

- **Social and Emotional Support:**

  - Communicate dietary needs with friends and family to ease social situations.

  - Seek emotional support from healthcare professionals or support groups.

- **Flexibility in Dining Out:**

  - Research restaurant menus for low-residue options.

  - Communicate dietary restrictions to chefs or servers when dining out.

- **Regular Check-Ups:**

  - Schedule regular check-ups with healthcare providers to monitor health and adjust the diet as needed.

- Discuss any concerns or challenges faced during the adaptation period.

3. Transitioning Off the Low Residue Diet:

- **Gradual Reintroduction:**

  - Gradually reintroduce higher-fiber foods to allow the digestive system to readjust.

  - Monitor for any adverse reactions or changes in symptoms.

- **Dietary Guidance:**

  - Seek guidance from healthcare professionals on the pace of reintroduction.

  - Include a variety of fiber sources, such as fruits, vegetables, and whole grains.

- **Hydration:**

  - Maintain adequate hydration during the transition to support bowel regularity.

  - Increase water intake as fiber intake rises.

- **Balanced Diet:**

  - Aim for a well-balanced diet with a mix of proteins, carbohydrates, fats, vitamins, and minerals.

  - Consider working with a dietitian for personalized dietary recommendations.

- **Monitoring and Adjustments:**

  - Monitor bowel habits and symptoms closely during the transition.

  - Collaborate with healthcare professionals to make necessary adjustments.

Transitioning on and off a Low Residue Diet is a dynamic process that requires attention to individual responses and collaboration with healthcare providers. Personalized guidance, regular monitoring, and flexibility in adapting the diet to changing needs are essential components of a successful transition strategy. Always seek professional advice for a tailored approach that considers both short-term and long-term health goals.

6.3 Working with a Healthcare Professional

Collaborating with a healthcare professional is paramount when navigating a Low Residue Diet, especially when addressing specific medical conditions. The expertise of healthcare providers, including doctors, dietitians, and specialists, plays a crucial role in tailoring the diet to individual needs and ensuring overall well-being. Here's a comprehensive guide on how to effectively work with healthcare professionals in the context of a Low Residue Diet:

1. **Medical Assessment:**

   - **Consultation with a Physician:**

       - Initiate the process by consulting with a primary care physician or gastroenterologist to discuss symptoms, medical history, and the need for a Low Residue Diet.

       - Determine the underlying medical condition and the appropriateness of the diet.

2. **Dietary Guidance:**

   - **Dietitian Consultation:**

       - Seek guidance from a registered dietitian with experience in gastroenterology or clinical nutrition.

- Collaborate on developing a personalized Low Residue Diet plan that meets individual nutritional needs.

- **Individualized Recommendations:**

  - Work with the dietitian to tailor the diet based on specific medical conditions, dietary preferences, and lifestyle factors.

  - Discuss any challenges or concerns related to the diet and explore solutions.

3. **Monitoring and Adjustment:**

- **Regular Check-Ups:**

  - Schedule regular follow-up appointments with healthcare professionals to monitor health status and the effectiveness of the diet.

- Discuss any changes in symptoms or dietary tolerance.

- **Diagnostic Tests:**

  - Undergo relevant diagnostic tests, such as blood work or imaging, to assess nutritional status and the impact of the diet on the body.

  - Use test results to guide adjustments to the diet plan.

4. **Educational Support:**

- **Understanding the Diet:**

  - Receive comprehensive education on the principles of a Low Residue Diet, including permitted and restricted foods.

  - Understand the reasons behind dietary recommendations and how

they align with specific
health goals.

- **Meal Planning Assistance:**

  - Work with healthcare
    professionals to create
    practical meal plans that
    incorporate a variety of low-
    residue options.

  - Receive guidance on portion
    sizes, cooking methods, and
    recipe modification.

5. **Supplementation Guidance:**

- **Nutrient Assessment:**

  - Collaborate with healthcare
    providers to assess nutrient
    levels and identify potential
    deficiencies.

  - Determine the need for and
    appropriate types of
    supplements.

- **Supplement Monitoring:**

- Regularly review supplement usage, ensuring that they align with individual needs and health goals.

- Adjust supplement plans based on changes in dietary habits and health status.

6. **Emotional and Social Support:**

- **Psychological Support:**

  - Address the psychological aspects of dietary changes, especially if they impact quality of life or social interactions.

  - Seek guidance on coping strategies and mental well-being.

- **Social Integration:**

  - Discuss strategies for integrating the Low Residue

Diet into social settings and daily life.

- Explore ways to communicate dietary needs to friends, family, and in social situations.

7. **Long-Term Management:**

- **Transitioning Plans:**

    - Work with healthcare providers to create a plan for transitioning on and off the Low Residue Diet as needed.

    - Establish long-term dietary goals and strategies for maintaining overall health.

- **Continuous Communication:**

    - Maintain open and continuous communication with healthcare professionals.

- Share any concerns, changes in symptoms, or challenges faced during the dietary management process.

Collaborating closely with healthcare professionals ensures a holistic and well-informed approach to managing a Low Residue Diet. This partnership facilitates personalized care, ongoing support, and the adjustment of dietary plans as needed, contributing to the overall success of the dietary management strategy. Always prioritize open communication and actively participate in discussions with healthcare providers to optimize health outcomes.

CHAPTER 7

Lifestyle and Practical Tips

7.1 Eating Out and Social Situations

Maintaining a Low Residue Diet doesn't mean sacrificing social interactions or dining out. With careful planning and communication, individuals can navigate social situations and enjoy meals outside their homes. Here are practical tips for handling eating out and social scenarios while adhering to a Low Residue Diet:

1. **Research Restaurants in Advance:**

   - **Menu Exploration:**

      - Prior to dining out, explore restaurant menus online to

identify low-residue
options.

- Look for dishes featuring
well-cooked proteins,
refined grains, and cooked
vegetables.

2. **Communication is Key:**

- **Communicate Dietary Needs:**

  - Inform restaurant staff about
  your dietary restrictions,
  explaining the reasons
  behind your low-residue
  requirements.

  - Ask questions about how
  dishes are prepared and
  request modifications if
  needed.

- **Advance Notice:**

  - When making a reservation,
  mention your dietary
  restrictions so the restaurant

can better accommodate
your needs.

- Some restaurants may be
  willing to prepare special
  dishes with advance notice.

3. **Choose Simple Preparations:**

- **Grilled or Steamed Options:**

  - Opt for grilled, steamed, or
    poached dishes, as they are
    often easier on the digestive
    system.

  - Request minimal seasoning
    or sauces to control
    ingredient choices.

4. **Build Your Own Dish:**

- **Customization:**

  - If the menu allows, consider
    building your own dish by
    selecting individual
    components that align with
    your dietary needs.

- This ensures greater control over the ingredients in your meal.

5. Be Mindful of Portion Sizes:

- **Smaller Portions:**
    - Choose smaller portions to manage the amount of food consumed.

    - Request a half-portion or appetizer-sized serving if available.

6. Hydration Matters:

- **Choose Beverages Wisely:**
    - Opt for clear and non-carbonated beverages to stay hydrated without introducing excessive gas.

    - Limit or avoid alcohol, as it may irritate the digestive system.

7. Pack Snacks:

- **Emergency Snacks:**

    - Carry low-residue snacks in your bag for unexpected delays or situations where suitable food options may be limited.

    - Nuts, rice cakes, or nut butter packets can be convenient and portable options.

8. Informing Friends and Family:

- **Open Communication:**

    - Clearly communicate your dietary needs to friends and family when planning social events.

    - Offer suggestions for restaurant choices that align with your requirements.

9. Plan Ahead for Events:

- **Potluck Contributions:**
  - If attending events where food is shared, consider bringing a dish that you can enjoy and share with others.
  - This ensures you have a safe and satisfying option.

10. **Focus on Enjoyment:**

- **Mindful Eating:**
  - Practice mindful eating to savor each bite and pay attention to how your body responds.
  - Enjoy the social aspect of dining out without feeling restricted.

11. **Stay Informed About Ingredients:**

- **Hidden Ingredients:**
  - Be aware of potential hidden sources of high-

residue ingredients, such as sauces, dressings, or certain spices.

- Don't hesitate to ask about specific components of a dish.

12. **Bring Dietary Cards:**

- **Dietary Cards:**

    - Consider creating small cards that explain your dietary restrictions.

    - Provide these cards to restaurant staff to ensure clear communication about your needs.

Navigating social situations and dining out on a Low Residue Diet requires proactive planning and effective communication. By employing these practical tips, individuals can strike a balance between adhering to their dietary requirements and enjoying social interactions without unnecessary stress or restriction.

7.2 Traveling on a Low Residue Diet

Maintaining a Low Residue Diet while traveling requires thoughtful planning to ensure access to suitable foods and manage potential challenges. Here are practical tips for navigating travel while adhering to a Low Residue Diet:

1. **Plan Meals in Advance:**

   - **Research Destination:**

     - Investigate the food options available at your travel destination.

     - Identify restaurants or grocery stores that offer low-residue choices.

   - **Pack Snacks:**

- Bring non-perishable, low-residue snacks for times when suitable food may be scarce.

- Examples include rice cakes, nut butter, or low-fiber granola bars.

2. **Communicate Dietary Needs:**

- **Airline Meals:**

  - Notify airlines of your dietary restrictions when booking your ticket.

  - Request a special meal that aligns with your low-residue needs.

- **Hotel Accommodations:**

  - Inform hotels about your dietary requirements in advance.

  - Check if the hotel offers in-room amenities like a

refrigerator for storing specific foods.

3. **Pack a Travel Cooler:**

- **Bring Perishables:**

  - If driving, pack a travel cooler with perishable low-residue items.

  - This ensures access to fresh foods during the journey.

4. **Stay Hydrated:**

- **Carry Water:**

  - Carry a reusable water bottle to stay hydrated, especially when dietary options may be limited.

  - Hydration supports digestion and overall well-being.

5. **Choose Accommodating Restaurants:**

- **Research Restaurants:**

- Look for restaurants that offer a variety of easily digestible options.

- Opt for grilled or steamed dishes with minimal seasoning.

- **Local Cuisine Exploration:**

  - Explore the local cuisine, focusing on dishes that align with your dietary needs.

  - Communicate with restaurant staff about your requirements.

6. Utilize Grocery Stores:

- **Grocery Shopping:**

  - Visit local grocery stores to stock up on low-residue essentials.

  - Purchase familiar and easily digestible foods for meals and snacks.

7. **Prepare a Travel Menu:**

- **Meal Ideas:**

    - Plan a travel menu that includes a mix of portable, low-residue options.

    - Consider items like cooked white rice, peeled fruits, and canned protein sources.

8. **Be Prepared for Unplanned Delays:**

- **Emergency Snacks:**

    - Pack emergency snacks in case of unexpected travel delays.

    - Non-perishable items like nuts or low-fiber crackers can be convenient options.

9. **Request Special Accommodations:**

- **Event or Tour Requests:**

    - If participating in group events or tours, inform

organizers about your
dietary needs.

- Request special
accommodations if
necessary.

10. Carry Medications and Supplements:

- **Prescriptions:**

    - Bring any necessary
    medications or prescriptions
    related to your medical
    condition.

    - Ensure you have an ample
    supply for the duration of
    your travel.

- **Supplements:**

    - Pack any recommended
    supplements to address
    potential nutrient
    deficiencies.

- Carry them in their original packaging for easy identification.

11. **Learn Local Food Labels:**

- **Language Considerations:**

    - If traveling to a region with a different language, familiarize yourself with local terms for high-residue foods.

    - This aids in reading food labels and making informed choices.

12. **Stay Flexible:**

- **Adapt to Local Options:**

    - Embrace flexibility and adapt your diet based on the available local options.

    - Focus on enjoying the travel experience while making

choices that align with your
dietary needs.

By incorporating these practical tips,
individuals can successfully navigate
travel on a Low Residue Diet. Proactive
planning, clear communication, and a
flexible mindset contribute to a positive
travel experience while maintaining
dietary requirements. Always consult with
healthcare professionals for personalized
advice tailored to specific medical
conditions and travel circumstances.

Made in the USA
Middletown, DE
22 June 2025

77368458R00057